EVERY DAY IS A BONUS!

KENN KINGTON

Published by King 2000 Publications. First Edition.

EVERY DAY IS A

B❤NUS

Enjoying the 3 Greatest Gifts In Life!

KENN KINGTON

Table of Contents

FOREWORD

I'll never forget where I was when I got the call. I was in New Mexico, waiting for my wife and sister-in-law to finish shopping at a lady's clothing store. The two of them had just been sucked in by the shoe section's tractor beam, so I was overjoyed for the distraction when I got a call from Kenn Kington's wonderful assistant Becky.

The shock came when I heard her horrible news.

"Wait, what?"

"Kenn's in the hospital, waiting to go in for quadruple bypass open heart surgery."

"Wait, what?"

"And his house has been destroyed in an earth-quake and his kids have been kidnapped by pirates and his wife has been abducted by aliens."

Well, that's what I heard, anyway. The reception

may have been a little spotty, but the impact was the same.

This couldn't be happening! Kenn's healthy! He's in shape! He's a good decade younger than I am! Do I need to go in for a cardiac exam?

I followed Kenn's progress over the next couple of days and was extremely relieved when all reports came back that my friend was out of the woods.

The reason I'm writing this forward is what happened a few months after Kenn's big event.

We were both in Nashville for a comedy conference and Kenn had been invited to give the sermon at a local church.

Kenn and I are both comedians. We've been in the business of making people laugh for more decades than I care to admit. But Kenn is a bit different. Kenn is one of those guys who knows how to inspire. Me, I'm always looking for the next punchline. Kenn has an instinct for going deeper. And on that particular Sunday morning, Kenn inspired me.

After the service ended, I told Kenn what a great job he had done and that he needed to turn his sermon into a book. Being who he is, Kenn deflected the comment with a humble, "Thanks, I appreciate that. It really means so much that you came out to hear me." At which point I interrupted him with a stern, "No, I'm serious. More people need to hear your story. You had a life changing experience and came out on the other side with actual *wisdom*! Whether you like it or not, I'm going to bug you until you write a book about it."

And that's what I proceeded to do. I wasn't obnoxious or anything, but any time we talked, I'd check in to see how the book was coming. Finally, this year, he finished it! I guess we have COVID to thank for Kenn's schedule opening up enough to afford him the time he needed to polish this off.

So sit back in your favorite chair and thank the good Lord He let Kenn go through his harrowing experience so that you don't have to. You get to grow vicariously through Kenn's brush with death. You have the opportunity to appreciate what you have now without going through all the invasive surgical procedures!

And when you're done, if you have time, please send up a prayer for Kenn's kids and his wife. Unless I'm mistaken, the pirates and aliens have yet to return them.

Robert G. Lee

INTRODUCTION

Not many people embrace change. It can be frustrating, challenging and hard to accept. Often, it happens when we don't want it or feel we can't deal with it. Yet, we usually find that in life, some of the greatest gifts, biggest blessings, and most treasured changes often come through trials. Trials test us, and often refine us. The unexpected situations and unwanted experiences often force us to places we would never willfully go, yet the transformation that can take place on the other side can produce a level of peace, thought, function, joy, significance, and true success. In short... a more complete and full LIFE!

While we do not always love what happens in our life it is even more irritating to be forced to deal with unwanted challenges! My life has been blindsided by a few of these unimaginable, unthinkable and very much unwanted experiences. While challenges can initiate great change there does not have to be a trial or trauma to bring about healthy change. This story is about one such life altering trial and the gifts that resulted from it. These gifts are available to everyone right now but it will take a reactive or proactive change to open them.

These gifts of great perspective came from the most traumatic physical challenge of my life. An unexpected storm that turned my routine world into a journey through the valley of the shadow of death in a matter of hours. This expedition was NOT one I would have EVER chosen, yet now possessing the perspective and gifts it provided, I would not trade it for a billion dollar winning lottery ticket. What happened in the fall of 2016 would move my understanding and enjoyment of life abundant to a level I could not have previously imagined.

I heard my wife tell a friend, a year or so afterward, "Kenn is different. He has always been a good guy but he is just different now in all the good ways." High praise from the one who has known me at my best and worst for over 25 years.

If you desire to experience the fullness of life, the time reading and digesting these pages will offer an opportunity for such a transformation. One does not have to endure a life altering, death defying blindside to gain such perspective. I guess I am just hard headed and it took that for me to discover the depths of three amazing gifts. I sincerely hope you do NOT go through the same experience. You can simply find a comfortable chair or pillow to recline with and enjoy the gifts without the tragedy. You will however, be faced with a choice to change. It doesn't matter if the prompt is a tragic forced expedition or a comfortable realization sitting by a warm fire. The best gifts in life are never fully enjoyed until they are opened! Experiencing these gifts is what causes the greatest change and most fulfilling difference possible. So what is this "difference" and how can it be engaged? Keep reading and you will discover!

QUICK TIRING
BACKGROUND

For thirty plus years I have done stand up comedy and public speaking for a living. I do around 100 live events a year and love what I do. No matter how much we love a job there are parts that can be tough or not the most fun. The most tiring for me can be the drain of travel.

A normal weekend usually includes a rush of travel. Up early to workout, quick shower and shave, pack and jump in the car for an hour drive to the airport. An airport can be draining in and of itself. Find parking, check in, security process, then get to the gate. Thankfully, Atlanta provides options for getting to and through the airport, but the mental gymnastics of it all can be tension-filled to be sure. Depending on the airline, the boarding process can also be an un-fun part of it all.

During the flight (usually 2-3 hours) I take the time to prepare some final thoughts or adjustments and review the ground transportation situation once I land.

Next, get baggage, get to a rental car (Shuttle or walk), then on to the hotel or venue. Once there, I usually iron whatever I need for the evening, take a quick shower to refresh and head to the event. A normal drive time to destinations is about 1-3 hours.

Although food is usually a quick bite, I make an effort to eat as healthy as possible. Grilled protein, salad or vegetable, nothing fried, and healthy snacks. Even if it's a drive thru I do a simple grilled chicken or similar, no fries.

Then the event details begin. Sound check, meet and greet, review the program with the technical staff and usually find a greenroom or broom closet (many times it is the same) to mentally focus, review and adjust to all the details of the evening.

The most fun is the event itself! I love encouraging people and helping them see the joy and hope in life! This part of the time just flies by and is why I love what I do!

Afterward, meet and talk with more people. I love people! Back to the car, maybe grab a bite to eat, back to the hotel, fall into bed around midnight or later. Wake up and repeat this cycle again for the next day or two. Another city, another flight or an even longer drive, and throw in some calls, radio interviews, check in with family, decisions about future events with staff, some articles to be written on a flight, prepare for the next event, etc.

This is the norm. If you are not tired just reading it, then please tell me your secret!

I usually arrive home after a few days of this rush feeling completely spent. I sleep in that first morning back to catch up on rest but still feel a bit fatigued. By day two I am back to about 90% plus and ready to begin getting ready for whatever is next. To say the travel part can run a person down is an understatement.

The problem was that I started to feel that "end of a trip" run down feeling during the middle of the week.

My initial thought was I'm coming down with something and just need to rest more, but that did not help. I was getting a solid 8 hours of sleep but couldn't shake the fatigue. I felt great during my morning workouts and for a few hours following but then just hit a wall! The fatigue started hitting me earlier in the day and just lingered. Out of a normal week I fought a mild run down feeling 4 out of 5 days. Then I started feeling the same sluggishness even on weeks I did not travel. Something was wrong!

AM I GETTING OLD?

My wife, Heather, and I had dinner one evening with a group of friends we call our Supper Squad. The ongoing fatigue was bothering me to the point that I decided to mention it to my friend at the dinner who also happened to be my doctor. I told him, " I know I have my annual check up in a few months but I have been feeling a fatigue for a couple months that I just can't shake and it seems to be slowly getting worse. I asked if I could stop by his office, get some tests and have him tell me that I am just getting old! He laughed and agreed.

After a few tests Dr. Cantwell confirmed my initial assessment, "Kenn, you are... OLD." Fifty-three didn't feel like I thought it would. It was nice, however, that I now had proof that it was normal and I should just move on. Apparently, this was my new phase of life. While I took the information as conclusive there was something that prompted my friend to offer one last idea.

Dr. Cantwell prescribed a scan. He told me it was around $100 and insurance did not cover it. He went on to say that there are ten factors to qualify to get the scan and I did not have any of them. I did not qualify BUT he would prescribe it if I wanted the peace of mind it might provide. For a hundred bucks I was all in! I wanted a doctor's opinion and a piece of paper that said, "You are fine!"

The scan took about 15 minutes total, and was simple and painless. I was told the test range for the calcification scan went as follows: 1-6 was okay, 7-12 was caution but nothing to fret over, 13-20 was a red flag and you need to go see a cardiologist as soon as possible. I left the scan facility with no worry at all. They mentioned they would let my doctor know the results within a couple weeks. Out of sight, out of mind.

The fatigue continued but I just figured it was part of getting old. I had never been old so I began to mentally adapt and figure out how to fix it with adjustments to my workouts and even more strict diet. Then I received a phone call...

SO I'M DEAD AND JUST DON'T KNOW IT?

I was backstage at a sold-out comedy show in Birmingham, Alabama. Minutes prior to walking on stage to perform, my phone rang. It's not normal to have your doctor call at night but as I mentioned before, Ryan Cantwell, MD, is more than a doctor; he is a friend. I'm very thankful for the many friends that would be pivotal through this life-changing endeavor but none more than him.

I answered my phone, "Hey Ryan!"

Since I had the scan a week or so prior, I was not thinking about the results nor what he was about to say. Our sons played on the same high school basketball team, and I simply thought he was calling to give me an update on the game. He was not.

After a few brief pleasantries he said, "Hey, I got your scan results back. Do you want to hear what they found? " I said, "Sure!" He briefly reminded me of the 1-20 scale emphasizing the 20 as the "BAD" end of the spectrum. I interrupted to give him an assurance I was OK with any result. I just wanted to know. So I thought.

I said, "I guess since you're calling this late in the evening right before a show, my score must be 19 or 20." He immediately said, "No," and I thought, "Oh Good!" Then he finished, "Yours is 697."

"697? I thought you said 20 was the highest, the worst?" I replied.

He said, "It is."

Confused, I asked, "So I'm dead and just don't know it?" My mind did the quick math and I thought, I'm 34 times worse than the worst heart? Take the worst 34 people with the worst scan scores and I am all those wrapped into one? My mind was swimming. More like drowning. Ryan then asked if I wanted him to read the lab comments from the test. I immediately said, "Yes" thinking it would give some relief or insight as to why this test was so far off and shed a little light in this very dark moment.

Ryan simply read the lab comments, "This heart is in the bottom 98% of all hearts (worst 2%); a cardiac episode is imminent."

Pause for a minute and imagine if you had just been given that news. What would you do?

I asked if I needed to call an ambulance or go

straight to the ER. I inquired, "What does this mean?" My friend replied in comfort and assurance, and I needed both more than anything in that moment. He told me he was going to check with the lab to confirm the results but that I would be fine. Just see a cardiologist when I get home from the tour. I said thank you and hung up.

Now, try and go be funny after that news! I literally walked on stage about 10 minutes later, did my set, went backstage and laid on a couch in the green room. I texted Dr. Cantwell and asked him to recommend a cardiologist, closed my eyes, and tried to wrap my mind around it all.

> *Even in the midst of darkness, I know God has an outlandish sense of humor.*

I called my wife, Heather, and shared the news. She had as many questions as I did but was amazingly calm. I expected panic and gloom. I got neither. My bride of 22 years simply asked what Ryan had recommended, offered to track down a cardiologist, and informed me she had been praying for this. Not for me to have a horrible scan but for progress, for insight and for an explanation of the fatigue I had been experiencing.

I mentioned that Ryan was going to text me a recommendation, and I would make the appointment as soon as I got home.

Even in the midst of darkness, I know God has an outlandish sense of humor. Ryan texted me the referral to the cardiologist, Dr. S. Manino. But, as I read the text I started to laugh. Not because of the name but because obviously his phone had auto corrected the cardiologist's name. The text came through, "There is a great group here at the hospital and I've heard **Dr. Minion** is really good.

"Dr. Minion!?!?" He wants me to go to a little yellow guy with one eye?

I can't wait.

4

APPOINTMENT WITH A MINION

D r. Minion, as I like to call him, was a great guy and full of energy. I called his office with my test results and the recommendation from Dr. Cantwell and figured they would rush me in given the stunning nature of my scan number. I felt an urgency to have this issue investigated, evaluated, and resolved as soon as possible. There seemed to be no rush on the side of their administration. It would be two weeks before they could fit me in for an appointment.

While that seemed odd, it also gave me a sense of calm. If it is not a big deal to them, why should I worry? My ongoing fatigue continued to ebb and flow. I figured I would simply continue my regular routine.

I had been eating a very healthy diet for a couple

years. Before that I had eaten what I consider a normal diet. It was better than most people but not super strict. I had not eaten a lot of fried foods for years. I ate very few carbohydrates. I had protein smoothies on occasion and usually a cheat day once every week or so to indulge in my personal favorite - PIZZA.

I worked out 5 times a week. Mostly cardio. I played basketball once or twice a week for a couple hours, ran on the other days (3-5 miles), and played tennis on top of the regular workouts. Basically, I was above average active.

I was 5'11", weighed 187 with no overtly bad habits. I've never smoked, never acquired a taste for beer, shared a glass of wine with my wife once every 6 months or so along with a nice dessert a couple times a month. I don't even drink coffee. My only dietary vice, I guess, was that I drank a ton of unsweetened iced tea. I gave up sugar about ten years prior.

People often ask me for the symptoms, my history, and why it happened. The only other factor that could play into the issue was a hereditarily high (bad) cholesterol. While I had high cholesterol, it had been under control for years with medication and diet. I had been at a better than average level for a couple years when all this happened.

When I finally met Dr. Salvador Manino, I was

even more encouraged. I sat on a table in Dr. Manino's office as he looked at the scan results and then at me. Back at the results and back at me. A confused look on his face was followed by shaking his head. I asked, "What's that look for?" He said, "This makes no sense. I have *never* seen a number this high. The lab confirmed it is correct but look at you. If you have a number like this you should weigh 500 lbs., be a chain smoker and an alcoholic." I smiled and confirmed, "Yet, I am not." Then he grinned and playfully insulted me with a smirk, "Yeah, you even look like you MIGHT work out." I laughed and said, "What do you mean, *might* work out!?"

He then began to try to discern the cause. Why was this scan so high? Why the fatigue? Why did this apparently healthy man have the results of a case on the verge of cardiac devastation? He tried to explain a few potential options based on the test results and informed me there needed to be more tests to figure all this out.

So I went in for more tests over the next couple weeks. The fatigue seemed better but it was still there. During and after workouts was the only time I felt completely good, even great. I felt... normal.

That reality confused the circumstances even more in Dr. Manino's evaluation. If there was a heart issue, working out should make it worse. Blood tests on several levels all came back in the desirable range. EKG heart rhythm was spot on. Great! So as a natural progression or last result, he scheduled a stress test with an ultrasound echo. I cannot remember ever having a stress test. After this one, I will never forget it.

5

JUST RELAX!!!

Tuesday, November 1st, I started with my normal routine. I got up early, rode my bike to the YMCA (half a mile), did a light lift and a 3-mile run, and rode my bike back home to cool down. I planned and prepared for the engagements/shows coming up that weekend and met a good friend for lunch. I was looking forward to dinner with my wife and another couple we had been trying to connect with for weeks. But first, I had this stress test to finish. The appointment was at 3:30 and wasn't supposed to take more than 45 minutes.

A team of technicians and nurses was on hand for my routine test. The treadmill was ready as was I. They hooked up the obligatory monitoring stickers on my chest and the treadmill began. The staff informed me that they would probably have to increase both the speed and incline a few times to get my heart rate up to the needed level. Once my heart rate reached a workout level, I was to hop off and lay still to get an echo of my heart. That's when it all started to go south.

I did my part and barely broke a sweat. I hopped on the table and just chilled. The technician almost immediately began to change the tone in her voice. She called over a nurse and they began quizzing me with intensity. "What kind of pain are you in right now?"

I replied very relaxed, "None."

Their intensity increased to a level just under panic, "On a scale of 1-10, 10 being the worst, how much pain are you in?"

I replied calmly and comfortably, "Zero."

I'll never forget how the nurse sharply snapped back, "That's not possible! Just relax, just relax!" Her tone was not comforting. It was fear, panic, and distress all wrapped into one.

I told her, "I was relaxed until you started talking like that."

She quickly sent for the doctor and kept looking at me in confusion. The monitor was telling her something was very wrong, yet the patient, me, was not at all acting accordingly given the indications on the monitors.

They offered to get me some water and moved me

to another room while they consulted with the doctor. The gravity of the situation began to set in and mental anguish started to consume my mind. God knew I needed a little comic relief in the midst of that stress-filled moment. The severity of the situation would soon be explained but I just needed a small break in the unexpected tension. And I got it.

What happened next was nothing short of a gift. A pause in the midst of chaos. I was sitting alone in an exam room for a couple minutes, a nurse's aide came in to sit with me and keep track of my vital signs.

She rushed in the room with deep concern on her face, saw me, then literally shook her head as if she was in the wrong room. Looking at her chart and the room number posted at the door, she confirmed I was the right person then released the tension on her face. What followed was exactly what I needed.

She smirked, "They're running around like you are about to die or something!" Then she laughed. I'm not saying she was an angel. I'm just saying I needed to hear her sarcasm and have a laugh at that exact moment. Her evaluation of the chaos was mine as well. I felt fine. Why are all these people acting like it's an emergency? We laughed. She took my vitals and she said, "I don't get what they are so uptight about. You're fine."

Fine is a relative term. What she and I did not know was the reality that had been eluding everyone. Dr. Manino came into the room, flipped on a screen, and showed me the ultrasound echo of my heart from the stress test. I am not a doctor, but it was not hard to see on the video of my heart there was something seriously wrong. My heart was convulsing and struggling like it was in great distress. Then Dr. Manino confirmed my observation. "Kenn, there is something seriously wrong with your heart and we need to do something immediately!" Those words still ring in my ears. As the doctor said those words, and I saw what was on the screen, it was the only conclusion that could be drawn.

Slightly stunned yet resolved, I asked, "How immediately?" He informed me that once my vitals had returned to normal, I would be allowed to go spend the night at home. He then asked what I was doing the next morning. I immediately asked, "What are you doing?" The doctor said he would be at the hospital and wanted to do a catheter through one of my arteries and look inside my heart. He said he would be there around 9:30 am. I informed him I would be there at 9:00!

We discussed the procedure and he shared two options. Dr. Manino said he hoped to find the cause and put in a stent to open the blocked area. He then introduced the second option. "Kenn, you need to be prepared. There is about a 30% chance you are going to need open heart surgery."

6

EVEN WORSE NEWS

The next morning the doctor and I were both upbeat. Let's do this. Figure out what's wrong and fix it. The procedure was explained, I was prepped, and he was optimistic. A short procedure and I would rest a couple days and be back to a normal schedule.

I woke up only 45 minutes after being put under for the procedure. The first words I heard were words you never want to hear from a cardiologist, "I'm sorry, there is nothing I can do..."

What was supposed to be a simple routine catheter and maybe placements of a couple stents to open arteries was now going to be the worst case scenario. I was told I was being moved upstairs to the Cardiac Care Unit (CCU) and placed on a list for immediate open heart surgery. An hour or so later, they started the process of preparing me. The gravity of the situation hit me in an odd way. It also had an effect on my wife that was equally stunning. She was not worried, not panicked, just resolved. At least that is what she showed on the outside.

> *The first words I heard were words you never want to hear from a cardiologist, "I'm sorry, there is nothing I can do."*

If I can be candid about my wife for a moment, she is one of those people you do not need to wonder what she is thinking or feeling. She wears it on her entire being. She is the person you want to tell any story, of any kind, because she will respond by embodying whatever emotion you might be trying to convey. She is completely invested in whatever you are saying. It is actually an amazing quality to possess and even entertaining to experience.

Next to empathy in the dictionary is her picture. When the apostle Paul wrote in the book of Romans, *"Weep with those who weep and rejoice with those who rejoice,"* I am certain God had given him a vision of my wife on which to base his admonishment.

My wife, Heather, is a recovering hypochondriac. Her motto in life for the first 20 years or so of our marriage was, "Worry early and beat the rush!" I have since learned this is a common condition of many moms. Yet, Heather was in THE TOP 5% of all worriers. She was so convincing with her ability to worry that if you listened to her long enough you too would begin to question your view of any situation and join in the worry. She has a contagious personality, thus my shock and confusion to her response at this life-altering moment. Heather's history of worrying early and worrying hard, and taking on anyone else's emotions made her reaction to this unsettling and terrifying news even more shocking.

She was completely calm! Stoic even. Unflappable. So if she was calm, my normal role, and I was on the verge of anxiety, what was happening!? It was unnerving and about to freak me out. Then she spoke of details she needed to arrange for the next day so she could be in the waiting room during my operation.

She told me how this was good news. The cardiologist had made it clear there is so much blockage that he could not put in enough stents to make a dent. I was in line to have quadruple bypass open heart surgery as soon as possible. Even in my mental fog I remember hearing, "40% chance..."

I couldn't remember if that was 40% to live or not make it but either way I was not particularly excited to literally face death in a matter of hours. So, why was she so calm?!?

God knows. He knows what we need, when we need it. As much as I thought I wanted some of that empathy and weeping, what I needed was a touch of rejoicing. God prompted that from my precious wife. Heather said at the pivotal moment, "At least now we know what it is! Now we can get it taken care of and   move forward." I felt like the universe had flipped and I was the one worried and she was the one just ready to fix it. Truth be told, it was exactly what I needed at that moment. Had she freaked out and become an emotional wreck, I would have stifled the emotions I apparently needed to experience and missed a critical part of the purpose of it all.

Heather gave me a gift. Assurance, clarity, and a touch of peace. As an extra gift, God managed the details of getting the kids taken care of and gave her time with them to prepare them like only a mother can.

Heather had just begun to pace in the hospital room trying to figure out how to get home to care for the kids and be with me at the same time. Grandparents had gone into action that day to pick up kids, feed them, and support the normal chaos that Heather handles flawlessly each day. She actually said, "I need to go home and figure out what they need and what I am going to do about tomorrow." Helplessly I laid there in bed about to give her my verbal permission to leave me and not worry about it. I knew she would worry and even try to get back up to the hospital again that night. Then the door to my hospital room opened.

SECTION 1:
THE
FIRST GIFT

7

STARTING TO GET IT

Ohne of the few moments of frustration Heather showed in my presence was the night before the surgery. I inquired as to what was on her mind and she honestly replied, "I need a couple hours to figure out what to do with the kids tomorrow so I can be here. I'll be back but I don't want to leave you alone." After a day of friends coming by and the weight of making sure "my affairs were in order," I was tired. I just wanted to chill. I was about to tell her not to worry about it and I would be fine, but then there was a knock at the door. Her desire to not allow me to be alone and my hope to just chill were answered at the same time by the same person. Dan.

What a gift to have friends that just know you. Warts and all. Good and bad.

Dan is that friend to me. We shared office space

and did life together for years. He makes me laugh and we just get one another. His wife and mine are identical twins born from different mothers, a few years apart but oh so similar in so many ways!

If there was one gift God knew I needed, it was my friend. It gave Heather the freedom to leave without worry and I had a friend to watch the game with and share some down time. I did not realize how much I needed that simple time until later.

We all need people. It is a basic need of our soul. Yes, we all have different personalities and crowds affect us differently, yet we need human interaction to survive and thrive. People are a gift! A gift we often take for granted. A gift I had for too long misprioritized.

I had a day full of interaction with so many wonderful people and it had filled my soul. My friends had come just to be with me. My genetically crappy and defective heart was full! I was happy but needed to recharge. A close friend who is one of the most considerate people on the planet was the perfect gift. The first of three life changing gifts I received from this experience was: PEOPLE.

People are a gift and are supremely important! There are so many wonderful people in my life but I simply remained on the surface with most and invested minimal time with too many that deserved more. Our culture impresses us to remain on the surface. Our pace of life can often throw us into schedules that force us to be superficial. The gift of human interaction is all around us but if I were honest I took little time to open this amazing gift and simply enjoy it.

I knew this in my head but I did not know how to live this revelation from my heart! Let me see if I can explain.

I am a nice guy. If anyone ever has an issue, I want to help. I would even have said, "If there is anything I can do just let me know." I meant it. The problem is simple. I never know what to do. Willing yes, but insightful, NO! This all changed. This experience has answered my ridiculously simple question. How do I open the gift of friendship and interaction and enjoy the depth of doing life together? The answer: be there!

Dan just showed up. He looked to see what needs there were and met them, even if it meant just sitting and watching a game with a friend. His gift of time and presence taught me and gave me a desire to do the same. I firmly believe it took being in an emotionally distressed circumstance for me to be aware enough to grasp this life changing lesson! I had to be the one in need of transformation into what God created all of us to be - people that care and choose to be there.

I discovered I had done little because I did not know what to do. I am a doer!

The revelation hit me that at times, if we are THERE and CARE that is doing enough. Mainly because that is what we all need. We need that basic support.

You may be reading this and thinking, "Kenn really isn't very smart or insightful." I would agree completely. But now, I have started to get it!

One of the 3 great gifts I received from this experience is this perspective of PEOPLE. People, friends, those who care and are there! That is the point. Not even what is done but just being there and caring. If there is an obvious need and we choose to meet it, then BONUS!

The most fulfilled and successful people I know in life are those who understand and interact with the reality that people are the purpose! It was Mother Teresa, the servant of orphans in Calcutta, India who was an extreme yet perfect example of living life to the fullest by giving this gift of caring for people. While living in poverty in the slums, she was surrounded by those discarded, helpless and hopeless who needed her and she never had a shortage of people to love. It could certainly be argued that Mother Teresa had one of the most fulfilling and impactful lives to ever walk this planet.

I had never been the patient. I rarely felt like the

one in need. I had never fully realized what it meant to be helpless. I had not been what Jesus referred to as "the least of these." I was the one responsible for myself and my family. I could always pull myself up by my bootstraps. Instead, I found myself in a position of complete need with zero ability to do anything about it. It felt horrible. What followed though was transformational.

I now realize the priceless gift of being a vital part of others' lives. Not for what they can do for me but what I can encourage, inspire, help, or carry for them! Jesus made this point succinctly when He said, *"It is more blessed to give than to receive." - Acts 20:35*

This was never more true than that night when Dan bought my "last meal..."

8

LAST MEAL... FIRST JOY!

Heather had hugged me and the weight of the circumstances had been lightened thanks to all our friends that had come by, texted, emailed, and called. And, at that moment, the tension had been wonderfully dissipated by my friend Dan. As we began to settle in for the evening and prepared to watch the 7th game of the historic World Series, Dan asked if I was hungry.

"Are you still allowed to eat?" he asked. It was about 7:00 and I informed him I had until midnight to chow down and I was starving!

Relaxed and informal, he said he would get me whatever I wanted. Then a wonderful slip. He started to ask what I felt like eating and sheepishly caught himself, "What would you like for your lassss..."

I started smiling and we both laughed at the gravity

and timing of the final word of his question. He was scrambling for a word he could replace for "last."

I couldn't help it. "Are you actually asking what I want for my LAST meal?!? It was exactly what I needed! Inside jokes, nicknames, shared pain, and joy are what life is about!

After a wonderful laugh, I had just given him my sandwich order and the door opened.

A sweet Jamaican nurse named Joy entered. T'was the night before the looming surgery. My friend Dan, having had a major surgery months before, understood what was about to happen. I did NOT.

Dan spoke with Joy for a minute and they determined her time with me would be about the same amount needed to go fetch the sandwiches we decided would be the best FINAL meal. He walked out and that is when my world would change forever.

Open heart surgery will leave a mark on every part of your being. Physically, it is painful in many ways. Certainly, the chest incision takes more than a little while to fully recover. Surprisingly it was not as bad as I had imagined it would be. The hospital staff had some tricks to help with that, including a heart shaped pillow that was a great tool to relieve pain. But your chest isn't the only part of your body they open up!

The leg incision where they harvested the vein to use in the bypass turned out to be one of the more painful experiences. I love the term they use, "harvest." In the operating room the next day, I planned to look around for a tiny John Deere tractor they would run up my leg to extract the veins needed for the bypass. As lasting as that pain was, it was still not the worst part. That would happen the night before.

There is an old hymn that quotes Psalm 30:5, *"Though darkness may last for the night, Joy comes in the morning."* The next 60 minutes or so would be one of the most dark and emotional times of my life.

As I sat on a hospital stool in my very revealing nightgown, I was already feeling a bit vulnerable. Joy, the very professional and kind nurse, who was there to "prepare" me for the surgery, sat in front of me. She methodically washed and began to shave my feet, then my neck, then up my calf and shin area. She moved up once again and shaved down my chest.

I should have put all this together at some point but she was so skilled and diligent it did not occur to me until about half way up my thigh... She is not stopping!

I am sure I blushed and my face was filled with discomfort because she paused to make sure I was all right. In a precious island accent, asked, "Are you OK Mr. Kenn?"

I said, "Joy, I am fine and you are doing a wonderful job." As my voice quivered and broke I continued, "I just need to close my eyes and find a happy place for a few minutes!"

She assured me, "I do this all the time and it's no big deal."

On the verge of tears from discomfort I thought, "It is to ME!"

This emotional procedure to eliminate all the hair on my body was by far the most painful part of this entire experience. I had no more finished the required antibacterial soap shower, dried, adjusted my sleeping attire and returned to my bed trying to warm myself under the paper thin sheet when Dan returned with dinner. I was still shivering from the shave and the required shower that followed. There was no hot water in the entire hospital that night.

Laying there shivering trying to recover from humility, Dan sat down quietly as Joy paused at the door. That sweet nurse turned and offered some kind encouragement and bid farewell with, "Mr. Kenn, I will pray for you!" What a wonderful gift. I wish someone had prayed for me before the shave but I'll take what I can get!

I said, "Thanks," and she was gone.

Dan, still quiet next to the bed unwrapping the sandwiches and securing the channel as the game began, started to snicker. I couldn't help imagine what was amusing. I asked a bit abruptly, "What on earth is funny!?"

His quick wit, flawless timing, and a twist of his head he said, "That's odd... I thought JOY came in the morning!" Such a rare and inside joke! He knew the same hymn from growing up in church and had held that one line for over an hour for the perfect time!

We laughed hard. I so needed that! The tension broke. The physiological pain floated away. Even the weight of the impending surgery and all the possibilities washed away. The Cubs won the 7th game of the World Series and I began to realize I had won one of the greatest gifts life has to offer... Friends!

9

THE GIFT OF PEOPLE

Watching the Cubs rush the field and fans celebrate what they had waited their entire lives to see was an awesome sight. It was also a simple reflection of what was my reality every day.

It sounds so trite. People are more important than fame, things, money, etc. We were created to be in community. Those long-suffering Cubs fans had one common need and after a century, that need was fulfilled. There was unequivocal joy. Their desire to be a part of that community was wonderfully overwhelming. People hugged total strangers simply because they shared a common love. In real life, I knew that and lived it daily in a very meaningful way. Yet, this heart experience punctured a membrane that had been keeping me from seeing the pure value of friends. In having friends, we love.

Galatians 6:2 says, *"Bear one another's burdens and so fulfill the law of Christ."*

Having people from so many different directions bearing MY burden just changed me.

I've always found great purpose and fulfillment helping others. Coaching kids sports, helping a friend move, listening to a broken heart, and thousands of other interactions. But, this was different. I was on the receiving end. While I had many friends share many experiences and give their time, support and lives with me over the years, I had never been helpless. Beyond an ability to immediately give something back, that helplessness put my mind in position to fully experience this gift of people and learn to both enjoy it and desire to replicate it once I recovered.

Romans 12:15 says it this way, *"Rejoice with those that rejoice, weep with those that weep."*

There were so many people who did so much for, and with me during the unexpected surgery and the recovery, that I cannot begin to keep track of it all. I want to name a few just to give you an idea of how powerfully their initiative affected me.

Jonnie W: I tour as a comedian and speak to various companies and groups during the year. As I mentioned in the beginning I am on the road about 100 dates a year and love encouraging people. My job has allowed me to meet so many wonderful people along the way. Jonnie W. is one such person. He is an amazing comic! The heart surgery happened right before I was to go on a 3 day tour. Jonnie not only filled in for me on that tour but sent me the check as if I had performed. Who does that?

My "Little" Brother: Family stepped in and was a critical blessing. They say the first day after open heart surgery is the worst day. I will attest to that! My brother sat with me the entire day and played goalie with visitors. He let me rest when I needed it and limited visits when I wanted it but knew when I reached my limit. What a gift!

Anonymous People: People allowed God to use them in ways I could only give Him credit. I was reviewing my calendar the day prior to the procedure and looking at the very busy month I would not be experiencing. One event in particular I had worked to secure for over a year and it was going to make my month financially. It was a big event! I was sitting in the hospital room a bit down over the payday I was not going to be receiving. My wife walked in at that exact moment having no idea what I was contemplating. Then she showed me her phone. Someone set up a GoFundMe page on my behalf. The first amount I saw gave me chills. It was for the exact amount I would be losing from the big event that I would be unable to attend. I still get tears thinking about it. God whispered in my heart, *"I've got this! I AM with you!"*

A Chauffeur: God continued to provide example after example of people gifts! Heather had mentioned to some friends that I wanted to perform at a show about a month after surgery and get back to something that felt like normal. The problem was I could not drive. No driving for at least 30 days post open heart surgery. Our friends Kim & Randy heard about it and took the initiative to help.

Randy, a successful lawyer and dear friend, volunteered to drive me to the show and back. An eight-hour round trip! He also had to act as road manager and did an amazing job! During our road trip he mentioned that his wife, Kim, admonished him as he left to pick me up, "Be careful! It would be a shame for him to survive open heart surgery and you kill him in an accident!" I love that many of my friends share my slightly offbeat sense of humor.

I could fill volumes with details of the hundreds of people I now realize carried me through one of the hardest times of my life. There are hundreds more I appreciate but will never be able to identify because they just saw a need and quietly met it. Christ literally walked me through the valley of the shadow of death and used so many amazing people to do it. I hope they all realize what a monumental difference they made in my outlook. I hope the realization that their action toward me has had an indelible reaction within me!

That reaction will continue to affect thousands that I come in contact with. It's a ripple effect.

> *I had never been helpless. Beyond an ability to immediately give something back.*

According to **Philippians 4:17,** the blessing I received from their kind acts that I now "pay forward" is credited in part to their initial act toward me. In simple terms, their blessing continues to grow and in God's eyes they continue to get credit for their initial efforts. It is a positive, eternal multi-level benefit plan.

A person's gift can only be fully enjoyed by being fully involved. Just giving to others will end up in burnout or pride. Just looking to receive from others results in an unhealthy imbalance. Yet being willing and taking initiative to give and humbly accepting help when needed is one of the most amazing experiences in life. These interactive relationships are more than surface or token giving and receiving, they are a transparent, genuine engagement. It is above circumstances due to the willingness to engage with one another in the process.

It has been questioned often, "Doesn't God want us to be happy?" The direct answer is "no." God wants us to experience JOY. Happiness is circumstantial in nature. Only when we have all we want, the way we want it and how we desire it will we feel happy. But JOY? Joy is beyond happiness. It is beyond circumstances and is experienced most fully when we are going through anything together, versus alone.

I can only begin to illustrate this amazing feeling through a real life experience.

We were in Costa Rica visiting friends who had moved there as missionaries. One day we went to visit some waterfalls. Hours into our hike to get to the falls, we were second guessing our decision. It was brutally hot. It was so muddy we couldn't keep our footing. We slipped every third or fourth step. We were gross, sweaty, muddy, and so thirsty!

Imagine the most thirsty you have ever been. Now multiply that by 2 or 3. I am serious. Stop and get that in your mind so you can fully imagine what happened next. Got that level of thirst and feeling gross in your mind?

After our two-plus hour hike of misery, the thick of the rainforest broke into a picture of perfection I had only seen on a movie screen. But this was real. A 30-foot waterfall pouring into a small pool then into a 40 foot waterfall with a crystal clear pool at the bottom.

Imagine being hot, sweaty, thirsty, and then seeing the most pure, cool, abundant water you can imagine. Now dive in!

We swam across the small pool and just stood under the pure water of the falls. As it pounded on us, the mud and sweat washed away. A slight tilt of the head and the endless supply of the coolest pure water on earth just filled our bodies. Just standing under the falls was like a full body massage.

Our souls feel that same refreshment of joy, peace, and hope specifically from the pool of genuinely caring people who surround us during life's ups and downs. If I close my eyes, I can still feel that cool, refreshing, life-renewing water. What the water was to my body at the end of that hike to the falls, the people who were with me, praying, helping, or just being there, during my crisis, were to my soul and spirit!

It was in the pain-filled, helpless place I would experience one of the greatest gifts that left me forever different. Shockingly it came through the person closest to me.

10

WHY ARE YOU CRYING?

I gained a new level of sympathy for many people, having gone through such an invasive surgery.

Ladies, I can now appreciate some of what you go through for beauty's sake that most men never understand. As I mentioned before, they shaved my body including my LEGS. Well, I now realize the fact that leg hair grows back. The prickly phase is just the worst! My legs would rub together in the middle of the night, wake me up and send shivers through my bones. I ended up sleeping with a pillow between my legs for a couple months for fear of the prickle attacks!

This situation has also allowed me to empathize with others in a variety of categories. I had a mild bout of depression for several weeks following the operation. Some would call it Post Traumatic Syndrome or

Survivors Guilt. The thoracic surgeon told me the massive amount of blockage in all four arteries was overwhelming. He said, "You should have had a massive heart attack 6-8 months ago and you would not have survived. You need to treat EVERYDAY like it is a bonus... because it is!" While full-blown depression is a completely different situation, I now have an appreciation for those who struggle with it that was not there before. I've also been given a frame of reference to both recognize it on occasion and come alongside some who struggle. I certainly don't have the answers for depression yet my heart has been expanded to care more for those who need someone to care.

When we realize life is out of our control, it can be freeing, but can also be terrifying. The discovery in this experience is that ...when we are at the end of our rope, done all we know to do, and are barely hanging on, it is not the end. It is actually the beginning of transformation!

...when we are at the end of our rope it is not the end. It is actually the beginning of transformation!

God continually uses these situations, not to simply build endurance, but to transform everything about us for our good if and when we allow Him to do so. It is our free will to choose.

I find myself much more compassionate and understanding. But the catalyst for it all came from my wife. She knows me all too well. This is the woman that years prior, during a small group told our friends, "Kenn never gets his feelings hurt, because Kenn has no feelings." She is not far off. I am a nice guy and very giving, but I missed the deposit of sympathy when God was putting in all the parts we would need. My motto in tough times was, "Just get over it."

That is until I wanted to get out of the hospital.

To be released following open heart surgery, all patients have to go through a class on how to recover at home. Many very useful details are shared during this class. Having just had my chest sawed open and wired back together I was not excited about sitting up in a chair for any extended period of time. So as the class lingered on, my focus on getting the material and getting out caused my patience to be in short supply.

The instructor stopped in the middle of one section and looked right at me and asked, "Are you okay?" I politely responded that I was fine and just focused on the material. She continued but clarified, "Not you, her," pointing to my wife, Heather, who was sitting next to me. Spouses were required to know the material also. With a quivering bottom lip Heather said, "I'm alright. Go ahead." The leader continued on through the next set of material, but a few minutes later she paused. Looking again at me she asked, "Are you sure you're OK?" I clarified once again I was simply gathering the material when she cut me off and directed her gaze to my helper. Heather was tearing up and struggled to speak, "It's okay, I'll be alright."

I was stunned and a bit put out! While I did not say it verbally I am sure my body language shouted, "What is your problem! Why are you crying? I have to do all of this and you act like you are going through this, not me."

While I have never heard God speak audibly, I have heard Him clearly in my spirit. There was no mistaking who was sending me this message, or what he was saying, very loudly. Paraphrasing, God firmly and gently said, "Hey Moron! She IS going through this! She is feeling everything you are going through. It's called empathy. You should try it!"

God teaches me so much through the precious gift that is my wife. Heather is Jesus with skin on to me and so many others!

Although I felt my heart grow three sizes in that moment, I will never forget it was later that night the lesson would be indelibly written on my recently reno-vated heart. God would use my greatest frustration from the night before to complete the transformation.

11

LIGHTS ON
OR OFF?

I f you've ever had any kind of surgery, you probably know this, but as I mentioned before the first day after surgery is generally the worst day. Coming out of 6 hours of sedation leaves quite a mental fog. Plus I had the physical pain that comes from having my chest sawed open, as well as the other excruciating details that go with it which are better suited to a medical journal (or a horror movie) than this book!

Just moving in any direction, I could feel the wire that held my sternum together. Then there is this new invention, a hospital bed that moves to keep sedentary patients from developing bed sores. I am not making this up and I was not hallucinating. Think of it as an annoying sibling digging his sharpest knuckle (times ten) into your back to irritate you.

It was constant! It wouldn't turn off. I was already seriously uncomfort-able, and this was the straw that broke the camel's back.

I woke up more than a little grumpy. I can't fully explain day one following the surgery because it was a complete paradox. I LOVED seeing family and friends and wanted to just be with them. I was excited to be alive and thankful for their willingness to come see me.

At the same time, I was exhausted and worn out. I was miserable either way. One clarifying example happened mid-day. The hospital has a program where they allow zipper club members (Slang for those of us with an open heart surgery scar) to visit new survivors to give a pep talk, answer questions and share a few facts to prepare patients for what is ahead. The two wonderful zipper club gentlemen shared some of the most helpful information I would later cling to. I wanted to hear all they had to say and wanted them to leave all at the same time. I just felt miserable.

I think I caught a glimpse of what my wife went through giving birth. During delivery, I couldn't tell if she wanted me to be right there and never leave or wanted me as far away as possible. I now realize it may have been both!

I hope this gives at least a small idea of how rough the first day was. What made it worse was that first night in the knuckle bed. My focus was on getting rest. I saw that first night as the finish line I hoped to reach. But it never really came. I had even kinda grown used to the constantly moving bed and blocked that out. I had heard multiple times from countless caregivers, "You have to rest! Get as much sleep as possible. The best thing you can do is sleep."

Take a wild guess at the only thing they do NOT let you do in a hospital? Sleep! After 2 to 3 hours of starting to nod off only to be awakened by another well intentioned nurse, administrator, therapist, vital sign gatherer, and other random medical personnel I realized, "I will never get to sleep ever again." Maybe dying the day before would have been better. There is not really a good English word for the combination of exhausted, irritable, uncomfortable and being in constant pain. If there is, I am certain it is a four-letter word!

The second evening was to be the turning point. That night I was fighting to hold on to my last few ounces of common courtesy. Conversations became increasingly short and my grumpy face and attitude were seeping through. Sarcasm was even starting to creep into my voice. All for good reason.

The hospital provided technically great service. While I never saw the computer screen the nurses, PAs, and doctors typed, I knew exactly what prompts were being filled in because of the repetitiveness of the questions. I could answer them before they asked and a few times I did. It was so predictable.

Right on cue that night, a shift change produced a new nurse with all the exact same questions. My saving grace would be the revelation of the last question that was always asked, "Is there anything else you need or is there anything we can get you?" I had cordially answered the exact same way each time, not wanting to be a burden on anyone. I guess in my subconscious I was ready to be a burden if it meant getting a couple hours of sleep. In a row!

The night nurse was a nice gentleman with little personality and very focused on his task. My guess is that he was former military due to the methodical and efficient way he did his job with minimal interaction. After the usual vitals and various tasks, he dutifully typed in the data and asked the final question, but this time my answer would be different.

He had shared his name and my short term memory had held it for this very moment. Before answering his obvious question, "Is there anything else you need or is there anything we can get you?" I paused. It must have been an inordinately long pause because he turned around as I contemplated how to phrase my request.

I said, "Dave, how would you like to be my favorite nurse of all time?"

He replied very monotone, "Ok, what do you need?"

I said simply, "Two hours."

He looked puzzled, "What do you mean?" he replied.

"I'd like to sleep for two hours in a row. Uninterrupted."

He asked with the same puzzled look, "What's stopping you?"

His question unlocked about 36 hours of discomfort and fatigue. I told him all about the parade of visitors from the night before, including the lady that came in to *weigh me* at 3AM... I think she took a wrong turn trying to find the maternity hall. He dutifully listened and my rant continued.

"Is there any way you can get all those people to come in now and just let me sleep for two hours in a row?"

He barely paused and with no expression on his face said, "Sure." Then he walked out of the room.

I lay there in the bed of moving knuckles and wondered, "Is he going to get those people?" Did he simply have his brain on autopilot and I sounded like, "Blah, blah, blah, whine, whine, whine?" The answer came even quicker than I had hoped. Within 5 minutes, the parade was back but this time it all happened in perfect symphony. He was a conductor guiding these artists to tune into my every need, test, and procedure. After a blur of activity, the room emptied. Dave paused at the door and with the same stoic, almost emotionless face he asked, "Would you like the light on or off?"

I sheepishly mumbled, "Off would be fantastic. Thank you."

I was awakened 3 hours later to a quiet and calm voice that sounded just like Dave. He whispered, "Sorry to disturb you but we have to get a few quick numbers. We will be out in a few minutes. Three minutes later he asked again, "Lights off?" I simply answered, "Yes, thank you!"

It was almost four hours before another soul would walk into my room. Dave quietly began the morning actively with an apology for having to wake me. Our conversation had turned... human. My frustration had swept away in the night and even *his* outer shell had cracked a little. As he went about his required routine, checking off chores on the computer I eagerly awaited the last question. When he got to it, I just smiled.

"Dave, I'm good! I'm really good!! Thanks to you. I just got almost 7 hours of sleep. I feel like a different person. You have no idea how much I appreciate all you did." He smiled ever so slightly and simply said,

"No problem," and scooted out the door to do his rounds.

I will never forget that morning. As I laid there, refreshed and contemplating what had transpired, I realized that night had been transformational. I had been transformed physically through the amazing gift of sleep. The realization that something else had also changed in Dave would greatly affect my life moving forward.

> *He moved from providing great care…*
>
> *to CARING.*

The hospital was an amazing place of healing with the best doctors and nurses. Their professionalism and service is top notch. But that night I witnessed something that left an indelible mark on me. Dave had moved. He moved from providing great care... to CARING.

Somewhere in that process I had moved categories in his mind from being a patient to being a person. I was now Kenn - the man that needed sleep and Dave had the power to provide exactly what I needed. He did not have to do it. He could have simply gone about his rounds and done his job and no one would ever know. But, he cared.

I'm not sure I had ever fully understood what that meant until I was the one in need. I had never been the patient. I am so thankful for that stunning lesson that every person needs someone who cares. Not just an environment of caring or an organization that cares, but a human. That gift would be lavished on me over and over during my time of need. I will never take the gift of people for granted ever again.

The second gift is intertwined with people in a way I had never experienced.

The best way I can describe the impact of the second gift in conjunction with the first gift is much like the relation of the ocean to the beach. Without the second gift it is like having seen the ocean but never gotten in it. To look at the beauty of the ocean but never experience it is to never understand the power it possesses. It would be like walking on the beach letting the waves lap up at your feet but never feeling the power and pulse as it moves you in the surf.

I was about to be overwhelmed with a wave of refreshment that would submerge me into joyful splendor. Time to take the plunge.

SECTION 2:
THE SECOND
GIFT

12

IS PRAYER REAL?

I t sounds so peaceful, gentle and mysterious. It often feels passive and can cause skepticism. No one really knows exactly how it works. I have struggled with prayer for the majority of my Christian life.

Why ask God for what He already knows and will give only what is best, when it is best? How does it work? Trying to comprehend the power and intricacies of prayer seems so overwhelming.

But, now I get it! I still do not pretend to fully understand prayer, but I get it. At least I get the foundational reason WHY and a major portion of HOW!

I have had a relationship with God since I was 13 and came to the simple conclusion that Jesus was indeed who He said He was and He did exactly what is written and was witnessed. I have experienced God's guidance throughout my life. I have failed so many times I lost count decades ago. But, I know what His abundant grace and righteousness **(Romans 5:17)** feel like and cannot begin to calculate how wonderful His applied truth has literally taken me beyond what I hoped and dreamed of seeing in my lifetime **(Ephesians 3:20)**.

Prayer as a part of life's journey was a struggle, sometimes sporadic and often frustrating. That is until I discovered that prayer was meant to be a multifaceted gift. Going through this traumatic challenge that could have easily taken my life was exactly what I needed to see prayer for what it is. Prayer became simple and clear during this critical time. Communicating with God and asking others to do the same answered two of the foundational questions for understanding everything in life:

HOW? and WHY?

The best way I can explain is through what actually happened. I did not know I was in an advanced level class on prayer but that is exactly what transpired. The paradox to it all is that prayer can feel like one of the most complex and difficult efforts. Yet, it is actually the most basic and simple form of communication in all of creation.

This situation all started in desperation as many meaningful prayers do.

13

THINK ABOUT ME LATER

My experience now is that God gave us this amazing gift to communicate directly with Him in whatever circumstance we find ourselves. Prayer is a validation and realization that we can indeed have a direct relationship with Him.

For those who talk with God and never "hear" anything I would ask a simple question: "Do you know Him?" Trying to pray having never acknowledged God personally is exactly like picking up your cell phone, start talking without ever having placed a call. It may look like a conversation but until we dial and hit send we are simply talking to ourselves through a device.

Until early November 2016, I was hesitant to pray with or for others. Usually I just kept prayers simple and general. I trusted God and prayed in conversations to and with Him but did not really "get" prayer completely. On that day when I was moved into CCU and awaiting open heart surgery, I lost all hesitation and inhibitions!

My wife had launched into social media to let people know what was happening. My wonderful staff had also sent up the flare to pray for me. It had come as a shock to many due to my seemingly above average healthy lifestyle and decent physical condition. I must say it was a huge encouragement that day to see all the responses. Hundreds, if not thousands, of people were texting, emailing, calling, sending smoke signals, all to let me know of their support and that they were praying for me. I can honestly say the peace and calm I did feel during that time surprised even me.

I am convinced God wants us to care about each other and to acknowledge that He is ultimately in control.

Prayer is a gift that has a couple purposes: It connects us with God AND with one another. It is an internal blessing that soothes the soul and spirit within us.

I lost all political correctness during my CCU day prior to the big event and prayer was the indicator. Most people echoed their prayers and support, but a few well meaning and kind people offered, "Hey, I'm thinking about you." I was shocked at my reaction and even more surprised by my freedom. While I could not respond to the countless texts, notes, calls and emails, I did personally reply to those "thinking about me." I politely and with a smile told them, "Thanks for reaching out and I appreciate your thoughts BUT pray for me now! You can THINK about me later."

My great desire was for this to work out for the very best, whatever that meant. I did not want to end up face to face with Jesus and have Him say to me, 'Wow, I'm really sorry. Nobody mentioned your name or your needs." My hope was the opposite. While I know we do not manipulate God and His will in this dynamic, ever changing world, the picture in my mind was having so many people bringing my name before Him, He had to cover His ears because it was so loud. I know from reading the Bible that God wants us coming to Him, asking anything and everything all the time.

WHY?

Because it is communication with Him. It is community with others, it is connection, and admission that we need something bigger than ourselves!

Does God answer back? YES! **Jeremiah 33:3** quotes God's best response to that question, *"Call to me and I will answer you and tell you great and mighty things you do not know."*

Now for anyone struggling or doubting that God actually speaks, don't miss the next chapter.

14

HOW TO HEAR GOD

S tarting to hear God is one of the most wonderful experiences on this side of heaven. It is indeed experiential. For many this explanation will confirm what they have experienced and it will validate how intimate God can and will be individually. For others, it may seem like trying to describe color to a person born blind but once we get the basic concept it becomes more clear with practice.

When we hear, physically, there are sound waves that enter the ear and move these tiny, fragile bones that create sound, and that is assimilated into waves that our brains then translate into words or distinct sounds. Make sense?

To hear God, it is the same process but the sound waves are not audible, they are spiritual. These "waves" enter, not the ear, but the spirit and soul. Just like the ear is trained by the brain to assimilate sounds and connect them to meaning, the soul and spirit will take the words from God and allow us to understand the truth. When we accept Christ as God and begin a relationship with Him by inviting Him into our lives we move from a dead, or dormant spirit, to having God's Spirit living in us.

To use physical terms we go from spiritually deaf to hearing. It is much like implants that are placed in the ears of a deaf person to be able to hear. God implants His spirit in our dormant spirit that is created within us. When we "believe" in Christ and accept His forgiveness and His spirit within us, we begin to hear.

The ironic part of all this is that during the turmoil with my heart, I realized I had heard God all my life since inviting Him in. I just didn't realize it because I was literally trying to hear Him physically. That may sound crazy but I don't think I am the only person who has had this thought. Don't judge me! Just laugh at me and know it's OK. Only rarely does God choose to audibly speak to someone. It really is so much easier to hear Him in our spirit as His Spirit lives in us.

One of my favorite examples of this revelation to me was immediately after coming out of surgery. Lying in recovery, the professionals in the room began to "help" me with what was ahead. I heard the voices of several nurses, technicians, and others. I was coming out of a 6-hour nap. I was in a fog. While attempting to get my bearings, the information was coming at me like bullets from an Uzi. "How do you feel? Can you sit up? We are going to try and have you walk today and we have some exercises for you to start." Then came the statement that would cause me great angst, "Kenn, you were on bypass for a very long time. Don't panic but..."

Anytime we hear, "Don't panic but..." is it ever good news?

The unidentified female voice continued, "Don't panic but you are going to have some level of memory loss."

The reason I discerned the next voice in my mind was God's voice was because there was no reason or explanation in my state of panic that I would have this calm and even funny response.

After anxiety shot up in my brain. I began to try and recall my wife's name, "Heather!" I rattled through my memory and named my kids, my address and a few other vital bits of information. Just as the anxiety had turned the corner to return to calm, my thought with an edge of anger was, I wish they had told me about the memory loss BEFORE the surgery. Yet, before that thought had a chance to take hold, a still, small voice, God's voice, in my Spirit cracked, "Maybe they did, and you just don't remember!"

I started laughing.

The pain in my recently sawed open chest was such bittersweet torment. Someone in the room asked, "Are you laughing?" I simply replied, "I'll have to explain later."

Yes, God has a sense of humor. By the way, God invented humor, laughter and comedy!

From my experience since surgery, I realize He has perfect timing too. We just have to learn how to listen. The more we ingest His word (the Bible) the more attuned our Spirit becomes to hearing His voice.

> *The more we ingest His word (the Bible)*
> *the more attuned our Spirit becomes to*
> *hearing His voice.*

A couple verses I had never noticed before this experience have become some of my favorites:

Isaiah 65:24 *Before they call, I will answer; while they are still speaking, I will hear.*

1 Peter 3:12 *For the eyes of the Lord are on the righteous and His ears are attentive to their prayers.*

As simple as this is, I am quite certain it may be too much to take for some long-time saints. There may be more questions than answers about prayer. This is my reality since sharing my story. Seldom do I speak that there are not some wonderful people that were a lot like I was before my transformation. The best proof in this clarity is that I feel zero need to defend what I had and continue to experience. God is never afraid of challenges and I have never felt the need to defend my experience. I do, however, long to clarify what happened whenever possible so others can experience this level of freedom and joy that comes with hearing God's voice.

While I am always open to chat about the details, I feel drawn to those who question the various aspects of the experience. Challenges do not bother me at all and are usually a great encouragement to both the person asking, and to me. I always learn how to better describe what happened and is happening when I'm asked to clarify details, or even when confronted.

15

ARE YOU SURE ABOUT THAT?

I had asked people to pray for me months prior to the surgery when the initial numbers came back so alarmingly high. I spoke at my church and told them the number 697 out of a possible 20, and in candid transparency, I told my friends and the congregation, "This is not resolved. I don't know what will happen. Please just pray. And they did! Weeks later I would go in for the stress test and consequently open heart surgery. They continued to pray!

I am a walking miracle, according to the surgeon and several other doctors that have seen the charts. I honestly don't know how one defines a miracle nor do I care. I live by the admonishment of the thoracic surgeon, "You need to enjoy every day like it is a BONUS!"

The power of prayer is as real as the mystery of it.

I was told on the day after the information about my memory loss, I would be in ICU for 3-5 days. Then I would be moved to a regular room for another 3-5 days. But, during lunch on day one, the doctor came in with an odd look on her face. She told me she was checking with the surgeon and my cardiologist but my numbers were abnormally great. It looked like I would be moved to a regular room that day, one day after surgery!

A member of the surgical team stopped by with a huddle of interns in tow while I sat in a chair enjoying my first real meal since before the procedure. It was just like a scene from one of those TV doctor shows. She asked the residents in tow, "Who wants to present this case?" As the white coated young physician read off my statistics the lead doctor abruptly interrupted and said, "Mr. Kington is a freaking rock star! You will never see numbers like this in your entire career. Let's move on." I waved and ate my pudding as the small herd exited the room.

About an hour later I left that CCU room for a regular room to recover - less than 24 hours after having open heart surgery.

The next day, while sitting in my new, less intense room, the lead cardiologist appeared again and with an odd smile on her face said, "We are waiting for one more test result that should be back tomorrow, but it looks like you will be going home in the morning."

A bit shocked I asked, "I thought I was supposed to be here 6-10 days?"

She replied, "The tests are clear that you are now where most patients are after a couple weeks." I offered, "I've never had open heart surgery before. I'm willing to hang out for a couple days if I need to. I want to go home, but I don't want to be at home and my heart stops or something." She smiled as she turned and walked out then simply said, "You'll be fine."

In less than three days following emergency quadruple bypass open heart surgery I *walked* out of the hospital. Slowly, but I walked. I've had surgeons ask for clarification on that timetable, "Are you sure about that 2 ½ days?" I simply say, "Yes, sir, I was home on a Sunday before the first kickoff!"

Prayer is powerful. While we will never fully comprehend its power, we can harness parts of it and enjoy prayer.

Prayer is not a chore to endure. It should be a conversation between best friends.

It is those that cannot enjoy prayer to which my heart is drawn to most. Prayer is not a chore to be endured. It should be a conversation between best friends. It's the place we can be most honest and vulnerable. That is why when someone is honest enough to confront any part of my experience, I tend to be most attentive!

The first time a confrontation about the prayer part of my story happened, I knew I had changed for the better and would never be the same.

16

I HAVE A BIG PROBLEM WITH YOUR STORY

Eight months after the heart reconstruction I found myself at a conference in the northeast. It is not unusual to have people ask questions or even demand clarification following a presentation, due to some of the spectacular details.

A young college coed was shyly waiting on the fringe of the crowd that had gathered in the hall outside the auditorium. She probably would not have even spoken to me had I not taken the initiative to say hey, but I could tell there was something on her mind. There was! Her first words, "I have a big problem with your story!"

The reaction in my heart was very new to me. I did not feel one ounce of being defensive or even being offended. Her demeanor suggested that she was grappling with something inside that I might be able to help with. I thanked her for being willing to come talk to me and asked what part or parts were so troubling. She dove right into the core of the issue.

Sternly she said, "You make it sound like if you get enough people to pray hard enough then everything just works out. What if we don't have enough people to pray or what if God doesn't answer the way we want Him to?"

That still small voice in my spirit was so obviously God speaking to me as she clarified her concern. It was not a reaction or a defensive tone I would normally have thrown back. It was a clarification and a genuine desire for her to realize the truth. It was simple and very brief. I said, "You missed the timetable."

Somewhat confused, she asked, "What timetable?"

When I described all those praying for me and the verses of truth people had given me and all the support I experienced, I did indeed have a peace I cannot accurately describe with my vocabulary. *But, it was before!* The complete peace was BEFORE the surgery! Nothing was resolved physically. I still had a very good chance I was NOT going to make it. I still had the same physical heart that the doctor said might not make it to the surgery, much less through it. Yet, the power of prayer gave me an unexplainable PEACE and calm.

There are very few times in my life I have seen a spirit right in front of me just change. She changed from anxious and almost bitter, to calm and even joy filled.

The powerful effect that ***people*** can create **(First Gift)** combined with the clarity of ***prayer*** **(Second Gift)** is taken to a life-changing level when the Third Gift is fully realized.

Effort and or desire to change is required to accomplish great feats. Or as the saying goes, nothing worthwhile is ever easy. These gifts have always been available to help us, but when we experience them working in harmony with the third gift, we move from powerful effort to effortless power.

SECTION 3:
THE THIRD
GIFT

17

GUEST AT MY OWN WAKE

These gifts did not become clear in a pattern but more intertwined as I experienced them and fully realized them by reflecting on the entire process. Actually, this experience was a culmination of clarification of these gifts from my life dating back to when I was 13 and began a relationship with God. If you remember from chapter 6, I was awakened from the catheter procedure and told I was to have open heart surgery. The time between that news and the actual surgery was full of these 3 gifts being fully experienced.

Those few days in the hospital were a blur and clarity at the same time. I know that sounds odd, but it is the best way I can describe it.

There were many kind words and prayers. The Two gifts, **People & Prayers,** began to synergize the circumstances away from gloom to hope. Yet, nothing comes close to the third component of this equation. The third gift is what pulled the other two into sharp focus and completeness. The first indicator of this third gift was a small gesture in the form of a text that simply caught my eye. In the midst of a vibrant room that felt more like a family reunion, with many of my favorite people, than a holding area at a hospital, this one gift stood out.

Then this third gift popped up in an email and another in a text and more and more. It grabbed my attention so intently that I would later that day crave even more. This gift did not detract from the people and prayers that were so edifying, but seemed to magnify those gifts and bring them to the point of a glow in my albeit defective, heart. That is the only way I can fully describe it.

These three gifts produced a sense of calm, joy, hope, and peace that words simply cannot describe. It was those amazing *people* and the precious *prayers,* changes, yet when partnered with the third gift: **TRUTH,** it becomes almost euphoric!

Caring People, Prayer and God's Truth seemed to be the perfect combination of all I would need. The gifts of people and prayers had carried me through so much of that day, but the final gift, the gift of **TRUTH,** seemed to elevate me to a higher plane, allowing me to see everything with a clarity that I think will take a life-time to truly appreciate.

As the evening wound down and the time for my surgery the following day approached, I found myself craving more truth. I sent out a text, an email and even a social media post thanking everyone who had corre-sponded that day and for the prayers. I could feel them! I then asked for more truth, "Please send any verses or passages that you feel applies to this situa-tion." Each verse or passage that streamed in was like another touch of hope. That night, after everyone was gone I read over those priceless gifts of truth several times. I read them slowly. I read them and the chapters in which they were embedded.

Shockingly, I slept very deeply that night but woke up very early the next morning. I actually had the thought, "I need to go back to sleep," and then laughed, "For what?" I'm about to take a 5-7 hour nap. Maybe I need to be a little tired. I picked up all those verses I had scribbled on a sheet of paper the evening prior and read them all again. While I immersed myself I would also gaze out the window. I had a room on the top floor of the hospital facing Kennesaw Mountain. The world was starting to come to life as the sun began to rise over the mountain. It was beautiful .

What the sunrise was visually, the truths that people had sent me were internally: calming, filled with peace, potential, and hope. The chance for a new start.

*In the beginning was the **word** (Truth) and the word became flesh (Jesus) and dwelled among us.*
John 1:1, 14

*Jesus said, "I am the way, the **truth,** and the life."*
John 14:6

Jesus puts it simply:

*"You will know the truth and the **truth** will set you free.*
John 8:32

The Bible tells us that God's Word is living and active. That truth written by God through about 40 different people on several continents over a couple thousand years is still applicable and alive today. What we read is meant for us personally and though it never changes, it constantly applies intimately and personally to any and every situation. The words will be the same, but the application and meaning will be what you need, when you need it. I realized how truth comes to us as I moved through this process.

18

LET'S GET REAL

How would you feel if you woke up tomorrow knowing you had a 40% chance that this is your last day? The real bummer is that you don't get to spend it doing whatever you want but are about to be put to sleep and may never wake up on this side of eternity again. But, there is a 60% chance you will wake up, so...

Let that set in for a minute. Honestly, how would you feel?

I am fairly confident no one can fully understand and answer that unless it is reality. I expected that reality to be overwhelming. I had gotten "my affairs" in order. I expected a heaviness of the situation to set in. The gravity of the matter was that I would close my eyes in a couple hours and when I woke up, the next face I saw was going to be either Heather or Jesus. A sobering moment to be certain.

Yet, something oddly wonderful occurred. It felt like a light, fun, easy day off. I had no responsibilities, nobody expected me to do anything except lie there and take a nap! That is actually what I was thinking. I am a simple minded person, yet this totally relaxed state of mind surprised even me.

There was zero heaviness. That morning of allowing God's truth to wash over the reality of circumstances had left me feeling cleansed and light! Verses I had read the night before and again that morning continued to echo through my mind; friends continued to stop by, text and email. There were even a few calls.

And, prayers! I smiled as I remembered Joy, the nurse from the night before, leaving my room and in a thick and distinctive Jamaican accent saying, "Mr. Kenn, I will be praying for you!" As kind as her prayer was, the experience from the previous night's preparation left me with one of the few side effects. Anytime I meet a woman named Joy I have an involuntary anxious twitch at the sound of that name! That twitch is the only negative result I can think of from this entire experience.

Others had stopped by to pray and visit. There were scores of messages from people who were praying for me.

The trifecta of *prayer, people*, and *truth* was better than winning the lottery three days in a row.

To be transparent though, it was the experience in the midst of it all that convinced me that these three gifts, working together, are the transforming combination in life no matter what the situation. It became reality several times in the days and years to follow.

But, the day of the surgery was the first and I will never forget what happened next...

19

I WONDER WHICH ONE IT IS?

E very time a heavy thought or the 40% chance of not waking up started to creep into my mind a truth would pop up and vaporize it like a villain in a video game.

"Cast all your anxiety on Him (Jesus) because He cares for you,"
1 Peter 5:7

That verse rolled through my mind several times. But no verse was more powerful than the one that flooded my consciousness rolling down the hallway toward the operating room.

Heather had squeezed my hand and kissed me for what could be the last time ever. Some really religious folks would not call what I was doing praying, but for me, I've discovered that simply talking to God in a friendly conversation is exactly that, prayer.

My conversation with the Almighty went kind of like, "Lord, I'd really like to see my wife again. I'd love to see my kids; to see them graduate, get married and even see grandkids maybe one day. But, I'd also like to see You! I'd love to have a body that is not falling apart; no more pain, no more tears. Thick hair again would be awesome too. Yet, I know if I don't make it You are going to take care of my/our family. I feel like I can't lose."

I quietly laid on the table in the OR and thought,
"For me to live is Christ and to die is gain."
Philippians 1:21

I get it now. I literally have nothing to lose!

Just then, one of the OR technicians asked, "Mr. Kington it looks like we are ready. Are you ready?"

I just sighed, smiled and said, "I am." I closed my eyes and went to sleep. I'm not even sure if I needed the anesthesia to get to sleep. But I did sleep, and time passed quickly. What seemed like five minutes was actually about 6 hours.

This next part is difficult to accurately describe. I guess you had to be there and I hope you never are! I began to wake up, but the process felt like it was happening in slow motion.

It was so quiet, deafeningly quiet! I couldn't even hear myself breathing. I tried to open my eyes, but I simply couldn't. I had the ability, but it was so bright my eyelids cringed shut.

Have you ever been asleep, eyes closed and someone flips on a light? Even though your eyes are closed you scrunch them tighter because it is so bright? It was exactly like that!! So quiet, so bright! So overwhelmed, I couldn't move. Then I began to realize, *I am awake.*

Scrambling to process the quiet and the light I started to laugh to myself, "I wonder which one it is!?"

I slowly started to squint. Anticipating, Jesus or Heather???" The light's intensity did not fade. I could barely make out the silhouettes and the quiet gently began to fade. As I blinked several times I could see a face... Heather! I smiled and started to say, "It looks like I made it," but something was hindering me. I could not speak. I was still intubated. So I flashed the sign for "I love you" to her with my fingers and after a quick kiss on my forehead, I was whisked off to recovery.

It was on that ride that I had another conversation with God. I was laughing. I am sure the staff thought I was loopy from the anesthesia but I was fully aware. I told God, "You could have really messed with me right there! I could have awoken a few minutes prior to Heather getting back there and some bearded medical technician leaning over me would have really thrown me. I could just imagine him saying, "Kenn, are you OK?" I would have sheepishly asked... "Moses? Peter? Which one are you?"

> *I HOPE everyone can experience such an intimate and meaningful relationship with God Himself. He speaks!*

Some people have a problem with talking to God on the level I have grown to enjoy. I could say on one hand, "I don't care!" and I didn't for a short time. That has changed. I do care and I care with the deepest hope. I hope everyone can experience such an intimate and meaningful relationship with God Himself. He speaks! He speaks through His people, through His word, and directly to our spirit that He plants in us when we initially surrender to Him.

In my basement at home, a few days after the procedure, I heard His voice - loudly and clearly, like never before.

20

YOU DID THAT!

The days following open heart surgery are painful. Learning to adjust to the discomfort was not initially easy. As I mentioned before, the hospital provided a heart shaped pillow to help. The instructions were simple. If you feel discomfort at any point just hug the pillow. Truth be told that really did work... most of the time.

Then I sneezed!

Crying from pain and not sadness was a new experience. If you would like to imagine the level of discomfort involved in a simple sneeze the day following open heart surgery, here is the best way.

1. Take any pillow
2. Hold it to your chest and squeeze it tightly

3. Now take a butcher knife and stab yourself through the pillow in the chest!

It basically feels like that.

I did pray after the experience and made a small request of God. "If that is ever going to happen again, Lord, would You be so kind as to please kill me right before that moment?" I have never endured pain like that before or since. I don't recommend it. If that was the lowest point in recovery, then what happened when I got home a few days later was a highlight of my life.

I set up camp in my basement. We have a very nice, finished basement. A big TV, wonderful recliner, my amazing in-laws allowed me to confiscate for a couple months, two bedrooms, the largest shower in the house and a kitchen. One of my favorite aspects of recovery was free time. Other than my breathing exercises and recovery walks, I was told to just rest and sleep. I attacked the breathing process which was surprisingly hard at first. The walks were a literal breath of fresh air. Yet the most renewing was my time to rest and ponder.

Each day I began by simply acknowledging the fact I was blessed with a second chance. To say I was thankful is an understatement. My thankfulness each morning was integrated with the list of verses people had sent just before the big operation. I combed over those verses again and again. I wrote them in a simple journal and even memorized most of them (listed in the back of this book). Yet, there was one moment that will be forever branded on my soul.

It was the first week home and I was trying to find the verse about "casting all your anxiety on Him because He cares for you." I couldn't figure it out from memory, so I flipped to the back of my Bible and looked up "anxious" in the concordance to give some guidance on where to find it. In the process of finding the reference in 1 **Peter,** my eyes were drawn to a familiar reference, **Philippians 4**. As I flipped my Bible open to the passage I began to read in verse 6.

"Do not be anxious about anything, but in everything, by prayer and petition."
Philippians 4:6a

The focus of my mind was immediately whisked away to the memory of the hallway in the hospital as I was rolled into surgery. At some point my eyes closed and I was there again. I could almost smell it. Then that voice in my Spirit revealed in a communication beyond words, *"Kenn, that is what you were doing! When you talked to Me about seeing your wife and kids and graduation and grandkids. That was prayer and petition..."*

My eyes opened in awe. Lord, that is so cool! I read on,

"by prayer and petition, with thanksgiving, present your requests to God."
Philippians 4:6b

Again, without realizing it, my eyes were closed and that voice as clear as a blue sky in summer said, "That's thanksgiving! When you confidently confessed your trust that I WOULD take care of them if you didn't make it. That is thanksgiving at the purest level." I started to cry tears of joy at a level I had never experienced. I am not emotional nor do I cry often or easily. This was beyond my control. But the best was about to happen!

With my eyes tightly shut and tears dripping I felt this joy-filled urge, "Keep reading!" I once again opened my eyes with a smile and tears uncontrollably mixed together. I read,

"And the peace of God, which transcends all understanding..."
Philippians 4:7a

Now the voice was coming directly from the verse itself. I'm not sure, but I think I said out loud in a basement completely alone but never alone, "Lord! I had that! On the operating table. When they asked if I was ready. That is it! Your Peace! I cannot explain it. Only You can give that kind of peace!"

> "The POWER of prayer
>
> is as real as the
>
> MYSTERY of prayer."

I was now rejoicing in a way I had never experienced. So intimate, so clear, so wonderful, but a few seconds later that voice slowly shouted in my soul, "KEEP READING!" I now had to wipe my tears and clear my eyes and find my place again on the page. As I read the next line I experienced release and was overwhelmed in the most amazing way I have ever enjoyed,

"And the peace of God, which transcends all understanding,
WILL GUARD YOUR HEART... and YOUR MIND in
CHRIST JESUS."
Philippians 4:7

Lord, You did that! You did that for me. With me. In me!

It was the greatest realization of God's living and active truth. I have never read scripture the same since. God has and continues to guide me with His Word. Those moments of simple intimacy when I read a verse and then hear the same verse from an unrelated source later the same day, or in a completely different context of life, are such sweet moments.

Some of my favorite times are when I come across a verse in my quiet times with the Lord. Later that day or week a friend will share the exact same verse and then again another time someone will pray and use the same verse. It is so common now I smile a lot and simply pause and thank God for reminding me He is right here all the time. How do I keep this going and continue to not only hold on to this gift of His presence, but experience and enjoy it continually? It's so practical and simple, so transforming!

21

TRANSFORMATIONAL RECOVERY

L ung capacity is drastically diminished after open heart surgery. When the therapist said you need to do your breathing exercises every hour, it seemed like such an easy task in the greater scheme of rehabilitation. It was not easy.

The small contraption had a floating ball that would rise as I inhaled. The goal was to keep the ball above a line marked on the tube for as long as possible. The first day I could barely get the ball to the line. I had to do that in several sets four times an hour. That effort wore me out more than the half marathon I had run when Heather and I were first married. This is to be done four times every hour. AND, walk 2-4 times a day for 10+ minutes. Just walk?

I attacked this routine as if my life depended on it and I guess it kind of did. I was told I needed to be able to walk one mile by the end of the first month and complete the breathing apparatus 4 times an hour keeping the ball above the line each rep, each time. That actually took me a couple weeks to master. I did feel better when none of my family could actually accomplish it and they were healthy!

The lung capacity portion was the foundation for the entire balance of the recovery cycle. Master this and recovery would feel like a downhill stroll. Blow it off and cut corners and the rest of recovery would be an uphill climb... in the mud... against the wind! As true as this simple admonition was physically, I can say the emotional and spiritual rehab was equally critical.

I did not know how critical until months later.

I had gotten into routines. My first was a simple commitment to, *"Seek first the kingdom of God..."* **Matthew 6:33**. I also try to remember this each day too: "Don't worry about tomorrow because today has enough trouble of its own. "One day at a time." Everyday really is a bonus and I was living proof.

At first I simply read over the many verses people had sent me during the two and a half days in the hospital. I moved on to reading one chapter a day where the verses were found, to get more of the context. I would take one of the verses and memorize it over a week's time. Memorization is not my strong suit. I wrote it down or marked it in my Bible and would read it out loud (by myself, in the car or shower) three times in a row and at three different times during the day. I found that by about Thursday each week I had it memorized. I also started to experience something... more.

I discovered each day while writing down my insights, personal struggles, hopes, and anxious thoughts, that the clarity of what I was going through along with the tone and pace of each day was more and more on target with where I should be. I found myself talking to God in my mind and heart during the day and picking up on other people's moods and tones and issues without trying. This emotional discernment was very new to me.

Also, my mood was so much steadier than ever before. My calm and peace were consistent and evident. Priorities and clarity were reaching levels I had not previously attained.

Was it the traumatic experience of the surgery? What was different?

I was ingesting the truth in ways I had before, but had never put together completely. This process was acting like an antennae, allowing me to tune into God's Spirit in ways I had heard before. I know this combination is the key for me, since I can draw a direct correlation to when I am actively seeking truth in all three ways, I am very clear, and when I am not, it is like a radio signal that comes in and out.

A. God's Truth FIRST. I want His truth to be the first thought in my mind each day. Before I look at my phone; before I talk to anyone; before I eat; before I turn on anything other than a light, I open His truth.

B. Read a chapter a day. Each day I read at least one full chapter of the Bible. On days I know I am tight on time, I may flip open to a Psalm and slowly read through a short chapter. Reading one chapter a day, I often read through a book of the Bible during a week or month. I highlight verses that seem to be speaking to my situation at that time. When someone mentions a verse in conversation, I make a note and read that chapter the next day. I was beginning to be amazed at how whatever chapter I read had a truth that seemed exactly applicable to my circumstances.

C. Memorize a verse a week. When reading a chapter each day there will be certain verses that stick out to YOU! Make a note and highlight them but also consider selecting one to memorize. There is something powerful about reading a truth multiple times during a day and allowing it to permeate our mind and soul. I've discovered the process of committing a verse to memory has multiple effects on us. Our sensitivity rises, our clarity crystallizes and our capacity for discernment heightens. Try it. I promise you will not regret it. One verse a week is plenty. Don't try to memorize a ton and burn out. Just enjoy the effect!

Conversations will be more meaningful and rich. Down time will be more restful and enjoyable. Everything will just be more joy-filled.

One day I saw it! The why! How it was happening and how it could continue after this recovery phase had ended.

When it hit me, I was alone and still laughed out loud. It was so obvious. How had I not seen it?

22

TWEETING JESUS

To get the full effect, we need to know all the components and a basic idea of where they came from. Trust me when I say we will want to know this! It is the secret sauce to maintaining the best type of relationship with God Himself. It's not the only way but it will be a huge boost of simplicity and practicality.

The overview components:

WE **time.** Years before the heart event, I was waking up one Saturday at home and mentally getting ready for my day. I was in that "not asleep, not awake" stage. The conversation I was engaged in with the Creator of the universe was refreshingly honest.

"God, I don't get prayer and I am really not good at it!" Why pray? You already know what I need. You are only going to give me what is best, when it is best. I trust YOU. So why pray?"

Then that quiet voice of the heart that speaks clearly asked me, "What are you *worried* about right now?" I was waking up and increasingly aware. My brain was starting to function enough to be clear, honest, and I remember thinking of a couple of issues. One was budget related and one was an area where Heather and I were not exactly on the same page.

Then another question popped into my half awake brain, "What are you *excited* about!?!" That was easy. It was fall and there were a few games I was looking forward to watching; as well as an upcoming golf outing with friends. And, a weekend away with Heather in less than 2 months. The things I was excited about were much easier to come up with!

Prayer is far more about enjoying an intimate relationship with the all knowing God, than making a wish list hoping I asked the request in the best way to get whatever I wanted.

Then that voice... "Kenn, that is prayer!" The realization that prayer is far more about enjoying an intimate relationship with the all knowing God, than making a wish list hoping I asked the request in the best way to get whatever I wanted. "What are you worried about? What are you excited about?"

Then came the goosebumps from that voice at the core of my being, "If it is on your mind, Kenn, it is on My Heart! I am with you!"

The reality is that the God of all creation desires for us to know He is always with us. Feeling our hurts and rejoicing with us in our pleasures is just what I needed. I have not been the same since. It is also a great way to connect with people. "What are you worried about? What are you excited about?" I will be praying with you on those and can't wait to hear what happens. I call it "WE" time. The world's shortest acronym:

Worried

Excited

The other components to this simple revelation of intimacy were also developed over time and have become a part of my daily ritual of getting ready.

Being Thankful. Starting my day with something I am thankful for is a regular component. Stopping and identifying someone or something or a recent answer to prayer or an attribute of God. Just being thankful gets my mind set in the best direction.

<u>Truth</u> had always been one of my favorite parts of starting my day right. Setting my mind on things above (Colossians.3:2). I listen to a sermon or in the course of a conversation with a friend or see a reference written somewhere. I make a note and read that chapter the next day and let God set my mind in a great direction.

The final component came after the follow-up visit with the thoracic surgeon. The doctor was very kind and honest in our brief meeting. I cannot begin to say how thankful I am for Dr. Myung. Did I mention I sort of lost all of my speaking filters during this time?

Dr. Myung said to me in the meeting, "Other than your heart, you are in great shape." Without thinking, my response was a little direct and caught him and even me off guard, "That may be the dumbest thing I have ever heard." Yep, I said it and couldn't stop myself even when he tilted his head like a stunned dog hearing a high pitched noise. He said, "Excuse me?" I quickly and gently continued while pointing to my heart, "If this doesn't work, none of the rest of it really matters!" He smiled and agreed, then I went on to say how much I greatly appreciate his amazing talent and for using it to save my life.

His next admonition was gentle but firm. He reiterated the condition of my heart prior to the surgery and the reality of what should have happened, "Kenn, there was so much blockage I have no idea why you are here.

You should have had a massive heart attack several months ago and there is no way you would have survived." He had my full attention. He continued with the final catalyst to my weekly day starter, "You need to enjoy everyday like it is a **BONUS** because for you it is!"

That comment stirred in my heart and mind each day until it became a functional part of my weekly prayer sheet. So along with what I am thankful for I list each day, "What did I **ENJOY** yesterday?" Just another wonderful reflection to direct my mind on the right path.

Each week I write a simple prayer using these components and one day it all came together like perfectly blended chocolate chip cookie dough - the right components in the right amounts:

Truth

Worried

Excited

Enjoy

Thankful

Each day, I write what is happening in each of these categories. What truth did I read? What am I worried about or what is on my mind? What is coming up that I am excited about? What did I really enjoy from the previous day? What is something for which I am thankful? This interaction has revealed just how intimately God is involved in my daily life. Sometimes it is me writing my feelings and thoughts and some-times it is what has happened in one of these areas. There is always movement and my deepest needs are being attended to.

At times I have wisdom and perspective that was not there previously. Other times I have a renewed strength to push forward. Then other times I have neither, just a sense of peace in the midst of the storm.

Power, perspective or peace, I find I always have what I need when I need it, from the ultimate giver.

I greatly encourage you to start TWEET-ing God on a daily basis. He will respond and it will blow your mind! Write it down or even better... Eat Jell-O.

23

JELL-O EATING

I like Jell-O and no I don't want to know what it is made of. It's fun and flavorful and enjoyable as long as you let it gel. Mixing the ingredients is important but letting it properly gel is what makes Jell-O... well... JELL-O.

It is the same with growing in a community and experiencing life abundant. Just like the ingredients of Jell-O we were not meant to do life alone. Also like Jell-O, it takes time to gel.

If anyone could have lived life to its fullest with no help and no support it would have been Jesus. Yet Jesus chose to surround himself with a group of men and women to develop a tight support system and caring for one another. He also cultivated the ultimate relationship that we too are offered. He referred often to God the Father, *"The one who sent me is with me. He has not left me alone."* **(John 8:29)** Jesus endured every feeling we would go through and He offers every human the companionship to go through it right along with us by living in our spirit.

When Jesus sent His disciples out He sent them in twos. In all of Paul's writings in the New Testament there are countless directives on how we are to interact, appreciate one another, and enjoy community.

I know when we are around people there will be some weird ones. Those that don't fit. That too, is by design. Jesus hand-picked His group and there was a weird one! Weird people teach us grace and patience and many lessons. If you happen to be in a small group and there are no weird people... then you need to realize **YOU** may be the **ONE!** Stick around. God longs to use all of us to help one another adjust.

If it feels odd at times to connect, that is normal. We are however, created to live in community. Help one another.

Rejoice with those that rejoice and weep with those who weep!

Romans 12:15

Carry one another's burdens...

Galatians 6:2

Take these three amazing gifts and live them wher-
ever you are:

Take in the **TRUTH** daily.

PRAY about everything. If it's on your mind it is on
God's Heart.

Out of all the **PEOPLE** in the world, you are the
only YOU God ever made!

Invest in yourself to be the PERSON God made you
to be!

Experience these gifts and you will discover the
abundant life God created you to enjoy! Start today
because,

Everyday is a Bonus!!!

24

VERSES FROM FRIENDS:

- James 1:2-4 James 1:27 James 3:17
- James 1:5 James 1:12 James 5:8
- Psalms 34:7 Psalms 23:3
- Psalms 34:18 Psalms 46:1 Psalms 46:11a
- Psalms 46:5 Psalms 46:10
- Romans 8:18 Romans 12:12-13 Romans 12:1-2
- Romans 8:6b Romans 12:5 Romans 12:20-21
- Romans 8:28-31 Romans 12:16 Romans 5:3-5
- Ephesians 1:18-19 Galatians 6:4
- Ephesians 2:8-9 Galatians 6:1a
- Ephesians 2:101 Thessalonians 5:16-18
- Ephssians 2:22 Hebrews 11:6
- Philippians 4:12b Philippians 2:13
- Philippians 2:13 Colossians 3:1-2
- Philippians 4:5

- Philippians 4:6-7 Colossians 3:23 Colossians 3:16
- John 15:5 John 16:8 John 14:7
- John 8:29 John 21:12a
- Jeremiah 29:11 Genesis 1:27 Deuteronomy 6:5
- Joshua 1:8-9
- Isaiah 41:10 Isaiah 43:5a
- 2 Chronicles 20:12 2 Chronicles 20:17

ACKNOWLEDGEMENTS

First and foremost I thank God for His grace, patience and mercy. Because of His truth, presence and patience I not only survived the valley of the shadow of death but have literally been transformed on every level.

I want to acknowledge those amazing medical professionals that without their gifts, dedication, and commitment I would not be alive today. Thank you for allowing God to use you so greatly in my life. It is because of you I have bonus time to enjoy. As a note, I have changed a few names to protect those who I had not noted during the process of recovery. Their faces and impact nonetheless are indelibly written on my repaired heart.

Those who were and continue to be such an intricate part of walking with me through this time and faithfully praying, giving of time and themselves is a blessing that is the catalyst to the transformation God continues to work in my life. Thank you and may God bless you and His favor rest upon you!

This book has been years in the making... While writing is not natural to me it has been a labor of love. The truth and "gifts" enclosed here are the result of several people's admonishments. Thanks to my friend Robert G. Lee who would not stop asking me if I had, "written the book yet" after hearing the story. Thanks to my friend Jennifer Carnahan who loaned her gift and training in professional writing to endure the major portion of editing. Thanks also, to Heather, Becky, Beth W., Dawn, Donna, Beth J., Brenda, Neal, Pam, Roy, Sharon, John, Brian, Samantha, Tim, and Steve who all took the time to read over these pages andffer much needed suggestions and grammatical transformation.

I am so thankful for my brother, sister, and mom who dropped everything to be there and care during recovery.

Words do not begin to detail the gift and blessing my wife Heather has been through all of this. I completely acknowledge that if there is any good in me it is directly due to God's grace and Heather's patience.

She sat by me and literally & figuratively walked with me in the hardest days of my life. Her effortless loving and giving heart makes my journey worth living. Everyday really is a bonus!

I love you all!

ABOUT THE AUTHOR

COMEDIAN

Kenn is one of the most popular Comics on XM radio, has filmed multiple Comedy projects that have aired on countless cable networks including Comedy Central, and performs regularly across the country. And, Kenn is so much MORE than a comedian.

MOTIVATOR

Kenn has spoken to Thousands of companies including several top executives at fortune 100 Organizations. He is finishing up his first book for the corporate world, "*4 Critical Decisions Successful People Make,*" and yes, Kenn was also a top 10 salesman in a Fortune 500 growth company before speaking and performing full time. His 2-minute weekly videos WOW Moments on www.KennWorks.com and LinkedIn (Kenn Kington) motivate and encourage thousands each week. But, Kenn is MORE than a motivator.

INSPIRATION

Kenn has spoken in thousands of churches of all denominations. Kenn has been featured on Focus on the Family and has written two bestselling books on relationships and records a regular video blog that inspires thousands to experience life to the fullest. Yet, Kenn is MORE than simply inspirational. Get ready to be entertained, encouraged, challenged and inspired. You will walk away with MORE than you can imagine...

Kenn and his wife of 25 years, Heather, live in Metro Atlanta (Kennesaw) Georgia with their three sons, and daughter (ages from 22-15).